I0503146

# Tips for ~~Surviving~~ *Thriving* Error, M.D. on the Internal Medicine Wards

# Mel Ona, M.D.

Tips for *Thriving* on the Internal Medicine Wards
ISBN-10: 1-4392-3124-9
EAN-13: 9781439231241
Library of Congress Control Number: 2009901969

Printed in the United States of America.

## Mel would like to thank:

Mom, Dad, and Bro (Eric) – for unconditional love and support

Dr. Giaccio – for guidance and contributing excellent ideas and tips
Dr. Martin – for amazing lectures and keeping medicine simple
Dr. Pannone – for mentorship through medicine and entrepreneurship
Dr. Munshi – for your editorial prowess and encouragement
Dr. Weiss – for reviewing my fledgling manuscript

**Special thanks to: www.BookSurge.com**

*This book is dedicated to my wife,*

*Jennifer*

*You are my inspiration and the love of my life*

1. Don't be late.  (*It's unprofessional*)

2. Be a team player. (*You'll find that work becomes more efficient rather than laborious*)

3. Visit your patients and know what's going on with their care BEFORE (not during) rounds. (*Preparation ahead of time will allow you to flourish rather than falter during rounds*)

4. Introduce yourself to the nursing staff and all support personnel. (*They will remember your courtesy and amicable disposition and be more likely to help you*)

5. Respect your colleagues. (*They're on your team and will support you if you show them due respect*)

**6.** Be sincere. (*Don't be a "brown-nose" – it's annoying, unprofessional, and points to insecurity*)

**7.** Document ALL encounters with patients. (*It's required*)

**8.** Practice, practice, practice your oral presentation skills. (*You'll be more poised and confident if you work at it ahead of time rather than winging it on the spot*)

**9.** Introduce yourself to the medical team: Attending, PGY-2, PGY-1, sub-I's, medical students. (*They will notice your confidence and welcome you to the team*)

**10.** Help your ward teammates. (*You may need their help at some point too*)

**11.** Allow others to shine. (*Your preceptors notice this and they will appreciate you for it*)

**12.** Say "I don't know" when you really don't know. (*Be honest with your lack of knowledge – it can be painfully obvious when you try to hem, haw, or backtrack*)

**13.** Don't be a "know it all." (*No one likes a "know-it-all" – check your ego and see Tip #12*)

**14.** Listen to your colleagues during rounds. (*Don't talk while someone is presenting during formal teaching rounds! Not only is it rude, but you'll also miss out on learning opportunities*)

**15.** Ask questions. (*You'll learn more*)

**16.** Don't ask questions that you already know the answers to. (*It feeds your ego unnecessarily and you're really not learning anything by doing so*)

**17.** Read 40 to 60 minutes everyday. (*Consistency is key to accomplishing great things – you can finish an entire 1000 page* *textbook within 12 weeks if you commit to reading just 12 pages per day)*

**18.** Visit your patients throughout the day. (*This will sharpen your clinical acumen – because you'll be more informed about what's going on with your patients and why things are being done for your patients – plus, it'll enhance interpersonal skills*)

**19.** Reassure your patients always. (*They will feel better and this is when healing happens*)

**20.** Be respectful towards your patients. (*You are a caregiver and steward of health for your patients*)

**21.** Treat your patients as though they could be your father, mother, brother, sister, best friend, spouse, partner, or yourself. (*Your personal and professional connection with patients is a uniquely privileged one*)

**22.** Smile more.  (*It puts others at ease and you'll feel better too*)

**23.** Be available to help your team.  (*Don't go home early just because you can – the team notices your efforts*)

**24.** Be present at all student lectures. (*You won't learn if you don't show up*)

**25.** Take notes at all student lectures and during rounds. (*Be an active learner – you'll absorb much more information and grasp the material more effectively*)

**26.** Read and review your notes from all student lectures and rounds periodically such as at the end of the day, week, and month.  (*If you are having trouble remembering what you've written, then you should be taking more notes and reviewing them more often*)

**27.** Accept responsibility for your actions. (*It builds character and fosters maturity and personal growth*)

**28.** Keep track of all procedures you've participated in. (*If something's worth doing, it's worth recording for the sake of learning*)

**29.** Read about diseases and current treatments at reliable websites *(E.g. www.UpToDate.com)*

**30.** Know more about your patients than anyone else. (*They are your responsibility and it shows that you are conscientious and that you care about what happens to them*)

**31.** Write down your own Impression/ Assessment/Plan even if you think you might be way off. (*This is where your analytical, independent thinking skills are honed*)

**32.** Think before you speak during rounds. (*This allows for more intelligent responses rather than hasty, unfocused guesses*)

**33.** Solve medical problems with a common sense approach. (*Keep things simple*)

**34.** Teach what you read. (*It'll stay in your brain longer*)

**35.** Don't make fun of others (*This makes you appear mean-spirited – rather, make fun of yourself as it puts others at ease*)

**36.** Sincerely thank your preceptors for their time and teaching on the wards. (*This simple gesture establishes a lasting connection*)

**37.** Ask for help during medical procedures such as IV's, venipuncture, arterial blood gas draws, NG tubes, etc. (*Remember to "do no harm" to others – if you need help, ask for it*)

**38.** Learn from mistakes. (*Fool your brain into thinking someone else's medical error was made by you…you will be less inclined to make that mistake yourself*)

**39.** Don't try to be "perfect." (*You'll frustrate yourself, and others, to no end*)

**40.** Strive for PROGRESS. (*If you can go to bed each day thinking that you improved at something or contributed to someone's feeling better or at least learned one new thing than when you awoke – it's a good day*)

**41.** Support those who are struggling. (*Helping others is a habit that you must cultivate because you have chosen a profession that demands this*)

**42.** Never accuse anyone of being a "poor caregiver" or "bad doctor." (*It's unprofessional*)

**43.** Offer solutions rather than complaining about problems you encounter. (*Winners aren't whiners and vice versa*)

**44.** Pay attention to what your patient tells you. (*It could be the difference between life or death*)

**45.** Respect your patient's privacy. (*It's what's right. And it's the law.*)

**46.** Spend time with your patient. (*Ask the patient if they have any questions for you before you leave the room*)

**47.** Introduce yourself to your patient by saying, "Hello Mr./Mrs. _____. My name is _____ and I am a ___year medical student who has been assigned to the medical team that will be caring for you while you are here. How are you feeling today?" (*Your patients will appreciate that you've acknowledged them first; rather than quickly visited them just to do exams and/or procedures on them*)

**48.** Observe from the interactions of others what patients respond to and what turns patients off. (*You'll be a more effective caregiver and communicator*)

**49.** Record your patient's vital signs and notice trends and changes over time. (*Be sure to let your medical team know of any changes in your patient's condition – it shows that you're reliable and that you care, and you just might save someone's life*)

**50.** Read your patient's chart…even if it is voluminous. (*Getting a full and accurate history on your patient reduces the chances that something is missed or erroneous with their care*)

**51.** Refer to your patient's daily medication list and note any and all changes. (*These medication changes may alter your patient's prognosis, length of stay, and general well being – stay updated on all orders written and follow up on them*)

**52.** Read all medical orders from most recent back to your patient's first admission order. (*This gives you a sense of the progression of care carried forth for your patients – plus, it allows you to pick up any duplicated or missed orders*)

**53.** Know your patient's past medical history and length of time they have had their illnesses. (*It gives you a more complete picture of their state of health*)

**54.** Know **what** medications your patient was taking before their hospital stay and keep track of all medications they are taking each day in the hospital. (*The more you know about your patient, the better you may care for them*)

**55.** Know **why** your patient is taking their medication, why changes are made (if any), and what side effects may be encountered with each one. (*Side effects can make your patients very sick – know what these are and* *how you can help your patient if these side effects become manifest)*

**56.** Read and follow up on all consultations in your patient's chart. *(Your patient's quality of care depends on coordinated and integrated hospital services and care-givers' recommendations)*

**57.** Read about your patient's condition in a classic text book like <u>Harrison's Principles of Internal Medicine</u>. *(You will remember material more effectively if you can make daily connections from the bedside to the books)*

**58.** Ask open-ended questions during your interview with each patient. *(It allows you to listen more and encourages open and frank communication with your patient)*

**59.** When a patient states that they felt "dizzy," ask them "What do you mean by 'dizzy'?" *(Allow them to come up with their own explanation – don't prompt them)*

**60.** Read EKG's on your own and discuss them with your team. *(It encourages independent thinking and analysis)*

**61.** Read X-rays on your own and discuss them with your team. *(It's great practice to exercise your 'clinical eye')*

**62.** Ask your preceptor (Program Director, Attending, senior resident, etc.) for feedback on your wards performance. *(You'll pinpoint your weaknesses – e.g. oral presentation skills – and be able to work on them more)*

**63.** Heed your preceptor's advice/input on how you may improve by APPLYING what they tell you. *(Knowledge isn't power…APPLIED knowledge is power)*

**64.** Write legibly. *(It can make a big difference in your patient's care)*

**65.** Work smarter. *(You'll save energy and stave off frustration)*

**66.** Maintain your energy by sleeping enough hours, eating right, and exercising consistently. *(When you feel better, you work better)*

**67.** Alert your PGY-1 and medical team about abnormal laboratory values or aberrant vital signs ASAP. *(Your patient's health and well-being are priorities)*

**68.** Go to bed earlier, wake up earlier and get to work early. *(You'll get more done and feel more productive at the end of the work day)*

**69.** Communicate with your medical team – ask how you may be of assistance throughout the day. *(Enthusiasm is infectious – spread it)*

**70.** Be an active participant during rounds. *(It shows that you care to be there)*

**71.** Know about *all* the patients on your team's census – not just the patients assigned to you – and be able to present them if called upon to do so. *(It keeps you sharp and you learn much more)*

**72.** Follow up on each of your patients (medical orders, procedures, lab results, etc.) in a timely manner throughout the day. *(Your PGY-1 resident will be grateful for your timely follow-up)*

**73.** Be inquisitive and curious about interesting or challenging medical cases – but treat each patient as a human being and not a "case study." *(See Tip #175)*

**74.** Acknowledge family members when they are present but address your patient one-to-one when caring for them. *(Focus on your patients and give your undivided attention to them)*

**75.** Know why your patient is in the hospital, what has been done in caring for them, and what your next step is in helping them become well enough to leave the hospital. *(You'll sharpen your clinical decision-making skills)*

**76.** Laugh with your patients. *(They'll feel better and so will you)*

**77.** Be patient with your patients. *(They'll be more at ease once they realize that you are there and actually care to listen)*

**78.** Don't cut off your patient when they are speaking to you. *(It demonstrates poor bedside manner and hinders healing)*

**79.** Give credit to your colleagues when credit is due to them. *(It's the professionally honest thing to do)*

**80.** Write your progress notes in black ink. *(It's mandatory policy)*

**81.** Sign your progress notes with your name, your medical school year, and your pager number. *(It shows that you accept responsibility and accountability for the care you provide – plus, it's required!)*

**82.** Stay in touch with your PGY-1 resident throughout the day. *(You'll find more opportunities for learning and helping the team)*

**83.** Meet with your PGY-1 resident before going home and ask, "Is there anything else I may do to help?" *(It demonstrates that you're a hard-working, enthusiastic student who wants to get the most out of your clinical education and experience)*

**84.** Make rounds with your PGY-1 resident on all patients in the morning before formal teaching rounds with the medical team and

Attending. *(You'll be better informed and prepared for Attending Teaching rounds)*

**85.** Have all pertinent laboratory values available during rounds for quick reference. *(A complete presentation is always better and more impressive than having to report that certain important results "are pending")*

**86.** Participate in clinical research during your rotation whenever possible. *(It'll set you apart from most other medical students)*

**87.** When making a correction in your progress note, simply make one strikethrough and write "error" above it along with your initials. *(It's mandatory policy and hones proper and legal documentation habits)*

**88.** Learn something new, everyday. *(You'll be amazed at how much knowledge you can accumulate over a period of just a few weeks with daily diligence)*

**89.** Review something you learned in previous days, everyday. *(Your recall will be vastly improved)*

**90.** Offer to assist with CPR when a patient 'codes.' *(You just might save a life – and this is something you will never, ever forget)*

**91.** Orient yourself to how a patient's chart is organized and keep forms and documents neatly in place (*If your hospital uses electronic medical records, then orient yourself to how the system operates – it'll save you lots of time)*

**92.** Orient yourself to where the medical supplies are stored. *(Be sure to take enough supplies with you and return the extras)*

**93.** Keep a "to-do" list. *(It builds your "daily discipline muscles")*

**94.** Check off all items on your "to-do" list that have been done. *(Keeping track of your* *progress builds confidence, consistency, and productivity)*

**95.** Keep a journal of all patients you've cared for. *(It's likely required by your school!)*

**96.** Discuss your patients in private…not in the elevators, café, hallway, etc. *(It's the law)*

**97.** Meet with the Program Director and Chair of the Department for input and advice on how to thrive on the wards.  *(They are excellent teachers and all-important resources)*

**98.** Maintain a positive attitude even when you are tired, frustrated, and stressed. *(You'll be surprised at how your positive outlook can uplift others who are just as tired, frustrated, and stressed)*

**99.** Stay away from "toxic" colleagues *(you know who they are)* and be professional always.

**100.** Don't take things personally (*remember that people are more than their moods*)

**101.** Write down all the reasons why you are committed to becoming an outstanding physician. *(The more connected you are to your vision, the stronger your commitment will be to accomplishing your goals)*

**102.** Ask the PGY-1 residents about their experiences as a 3rd or 4th year medical student. *(You'll often save much time and effort by learning from their mistakes and pitfalls)*

**103.** Graph/trend your patient's lab data. *(So you can get an overall sense of their progress and prognosis)*

**104.** Organize your patient's information in confidential concise summaries and files (*for ease of reference*)

**105.** Do your work carefully and conscientiously. (*and timely*)

**106.** Write thank you notes and give them to your preceptors. (*Be honest and sincere with your thanks – don't say you enjoyed a rotation when you really didn't*)

**107.** Read your school's Internal Medicine Clerkship Orientation Packet and heed all important notices, recommendations, and requirements on the wards. (*It's your roadmap that'll guide you through your journey on the wards*)

**108.** Be present at mandatory conferences. (*You can't learn if you're not there*)

**109.** Be awake and alert and oriented at mandatory conferences. (*Take notes – it'll help you stay awake and you'll have something to review afterwards*)

**110.** Shred all unused documents that display patient identification. *(Respect patient privacy always)*

**111.** Consolidate and group your lecture notes according to organ system or topic (Neuro, Cardio, GI, Nephro, Endo, ID, etc.) for quick reference and organized review. *(It will make your studying more organized and efficient as you prepare for Shelf Exams and the Boards)*

**112.** Be willing to observe and assist with procedures (e.g. triple lumen catheter placement, foley catheter insertion, EGD, etc.). *(See a few, do a bunch, teach as much as possible)*

**113.** Wash your hands with soap and warm water (and with the alcohol-based sanitizing dispensers) before and after seeing your patients. *(Hygiene tip: The best way to wash your hands is to wet them first before applying the soap!)*

**114.** Sing "Happy Birthday" three times slowly to yourself while washing your hands with adequate friction and with soap and warm water…that's approximately how long you should wash them for! *(~30 seconds – seriously, it kills C. difficile!)*

**115.** Gently remind your colleagues to wash their hands before and after seeing their patients. *(Spread the health)*

**116.** Use paper towels to turn off public faucets and to open doors before leaving public restrooms. *(The people who don't wash their hands leave plenty of germs on these surfaces)*

**117.** Have your stethoscope, penlight, tuning fork, reflex hammer, and alcohol prep pads handy. *(You'll find that you need them the most…when you don't have them)*

**118.** Wipe down your stethoscope, penlight, tuning fork, reflex hammer and other tools with alcohol prep pads on a daily basis. *(It reduces the chances of spreading disease to your patients or to yourself)*

**119.** Change your white coat on a regular basis. *(You'd be surprised at how dingy and nasty they get)*

**120.** Expand your differential diagnosis list while working up a new patient. *(It trains your brain to think like a top doctor who is always problem solving and thinking deductively, laterally, and analytically)*

**121.** ***DDx challenge:*** Try to come up with 17 differential diagnoses for your patient's chief symptom complaint. *(You'll integrate your knowledge of the body's multiple systems and how they interact)*

**122.** Study the differential diagnoses and standards of care for the most common presenting symptoms that patients come to the hospital for *(E.g. chest pain, shortness of breath, abdominal pain, etc.)*

**123.** Ask your Attending what they expect in an oral presentation during formal teaching rounds (E.g. how much information to give and in what time allotment). *(See Tip #8)*

**124.** Be an active participant during discussions with Social Workers and the medical team regarding discharge planning. *(It's an integral part of patient care – ensuring that they have someplace to go, which will support their recovery and well-being)*

**125.** Be *visible* and *available* to your PGY-1 resident. *(Imagine the type of medical student whom you would want to help you when you're a PGY-1 intern – be that student now)*

**126.** Meet with your PGY-2 resident for tips on how they succeeded during their PGY-1 year. *(The insight they have about the intern year can save you time, stress, and heartache)*

**127.** Introduce yourself to PGY-3 residents and learn about their personal experiences during PGY-1 and PGY-2 years. *(They have accumulated knowledge and experience that can inspire you to stay the course and strive to be the outstanding doctor that you know you will be)*

**128.** Focus on obtaining a complete medical history for each of your patients. *(A complete history makes your presentation more compelling and allows for optimal diagnosis - remember that 95% of diagnoses may come from the history that a patient gives!)*

**129.** Always think: *"What needs to be done so that my patient can get the best possible care and ultimately become medically well for discharge from the hospital?"*

**130.** Read a review book or do practice questions during "down time" if on call and waiting for an admission. *(Maximizing your downtime by studying will keep you sharp on the wards and build your confidence for the boards)*

**131.** Accompany your PGY-1 resident during Outpatient Clinic and observe patient care in this setting. *(It's a smart idea to see and experience the various aspects of what medicine offers)*

**132.** Have an organized format when presenting your patient during formal teaching rounds: An example might be: "This is Mr./Mrs./Miss ____. He/She is a __ year-old male/female who came to ER on ___(day/date) complaining of _____ (chief complaint). Past medical history is significant for ___. The patient reports _____ (briefly describe history of present illness including pertinent medications, family history, social history, contributory review of systems and physical exam). He/She was admitted for ____ and now the patient is _____(describe hospital course and impression/plan)." *(Keep it simple, direct, clear, and complete)*

**133.** Speak clearly, confidently, slowly, and address the medical team while presenting your patient during formal teaching rounds rather than reading from a script. *(You'll impress your evaluators and strengthen your public-speaking skills tremendously)*

**134.** Introduce your patient to the medical team if meeting for the first time: "Good morning Mr./Mrs./Miss _____. This is our teaching doctor (Attending) and we are the medical team who will care for you at this time." *(It shows that you are polite, conscientious, and sensitive to the patient's pivotal role in the learning process – all centered around caring for the patient)*

**135.** Observe and learn from the interactions between the Attending and your patients – taking note of what questions the Attending asks and how he/she responds to the patients' concerns. *(What better way to learn than from doctors who have many years of experience caring at the bedside)*

**136.** Read what the Attending writes in your patient's chart and follow up on any/all orders immediately after rounds. *(Whatever the Attending says or writes is what's to be done for the patient – don't delay necessary care)*

**137.** Call back right away when you have been paged. *(It shows that you're reliable and prompt)*

**138.** Be honest when writing progress notes on your patients *(Don't write "Lungs are clear" if you did not listen to them – even if a previous note indicated that the patient's lungs were clear…be HONEST always)*

**139.** Don't leave blank spaces when writing notes in your patient's chart – if you need to fill in missing information, write "pending" and then write an addendum (with date, time, and your signature) later. *(Blank spaces = poor charting habits…avoid leaving them)*

**140.** Seek clarification if you cannot decipher handwriting on your patient's chart – especially the medical orders. *(It could save or cost a patient's life depending on what's actually written vs. what you might interpret what the handwritten order says)*

**141.** Find out ahead of time what conferences and/or lectures are scheduled for the day so that you can read a bit about the topic before it is presented. *(Pre-reading aids memory retention)*

**142.** Write (or type if electronic) your progress notes in an acceptable format: E.g. S.O.A.P. = Subjective, Objective, Assessment, Plan and finish your notes as soon as possible after seeing your patients. *(It will* *enhance the timeliness and continuity of care for your patients)*

**143.** Keep your progress notes to the point and do not feel compelled to write pages upon pages about your patient. *(Stay focused and write the most pertinent and important findings about your patient)*

**144.** Be confident, careful, and compassionate when performing procedures on your patients *(e.g. venipuncture, NG tubes, arterial blood draws, catheters, etc. – tell them ahead of time that "you will feel a sharp scratch" if drawing blood)*

**145.** Prepare all materials ahead of time when performing procedures on your patients (e.g. venipuncture, NG tubes, arterial blood draws, catheters, etc.) including patient labels on tubes, paperwork, specimen bags, gloves, etc. *(You'll be more efficient and save time)*

**146.** When in doubt, ask for help. *(Ask nicely)*

**147.** Be proactive *(Not passive)*

**148.** Be patient *(Not pushy)*

**149.** Commend your fellow medical colleagues *(Don't complain to them)*

**150.** Evaluate your preceptors (e.g. Attendings, senior residents, intern) in writing - honestly, thoroughly, and constructively. *(Constant and never-ending improvement is the goal)*

**151.** Be polite and act kindly when making requests of support personnel (i.e. nurses, clerks, maintenance staff, etc.). *(They will be more inclined to help you when you really need it in the future)*

**152.** Thank your patients for their patience and openness in allowing you to learn from them. *(A simple gesture of thanks can make significant gains in connecting with your patients and helping you maintain perspective that you are both learning and healing at the same time)*

**153.** If you are assigned different patients or are switched to a new medical team, say goodbye to your patients and wish them well. *(They will never forget you)*

**154.** Seek mentors (i.e. Program Director, Attending physicians) early in the rotation and make appointments to chat with them or find opportunities to learn from them by asking questions. *(These are the same important people who may write Letters of Recommendation for you in the near future – get to know them)*

**155.** Make a list of topics that you would like to discuss during the medical student lectures and share them with your medical student peers *(Chances are they would have made the same list)*

156. Take notes about the process and rationale for why things are done for patients – tests, scans, procedures – and be thoughtful in your approach rather than robotically following a "protocol." *(This is where the "art" of clinical medicine becomes honed – you'll begin to notice patterns, problem-solve, and be able to justify WHY things are being done with your patients)*

157. Observe your Attendings take a history for patients and note the type and flow of questions that allow them to quickly arrive at several differential diagnoses, deftly make an impression, and logically formulate an effective, evidence-based treatment plan. *(One of the best methods of learning is to model the experts – do as they do and you will achieve similar skills in a shorter period of time)*

**158.** Ask your Attendings about past cases that challenged them and how they worked through them. *(It helps to breakdown how experienced clinicians logically think through patient care – especially with difficult cases)*

**159.** Request feedback from your PGY-1 resident regarding your history taking and physical examination skills. *(Seeking comments about your bedside manner and patient interviewing shows that you're willing to improve these all-important skills)*

**160.** Stick with one primary textbook resource (e.g. <u>Harrison's Principles of Internal Medicine</u>) and one or two review books for studying for end-of-rotation exams. *(Having too many sources – i.e. source overload – is counterproductive; aim for knowing 1 or 2 sources very well rather than glossing over 5 or 6 sources)*

**161.** Be professional at all times throughout the day…in the cafeteria too. *(You never know who might be sitting nearby)*

**162.** Before going to bed, read one chapter from a reliable text about the disease that each of your patients presents with. *(You'll remember details about your patient's condition and understand their care better)*

**163.** Be nice to all the nurses and ward clerks on the medical floors with whom you will be working. *(No one thrives in a hostile environment)*

**164.** Dress well for success. *(It fosters maturity and professionalism…and also, you are being evaluated constantly by your superiors, peers, and patients)*

**165.** Take a 30–45 minute break during the day to sit down, relax, and eat something nutritious. *(A healthy, rested and fed you is a more productive, energetic, and satisfied you)*

**166.** Stay calm, be cool, remain collected, and think "win-win" when faced with conflict (from staff and/or students) on the wards. *(It's better to be at peace than to be "right")*

**167.** Share ideas with your Program Director about improving any aspect of the clerkship – with humility and enthusiasm. *(Improvement in the system helps everyone)*

**168.** Chat with the Program Director and ask, "what attributes and skills enable a 3$^{rd}$ and 4$^{th}$ year medical student to become an outstanding intern and beyond?" *(Your PD is a goldmine of tips, strategies, and sage advice)*

**169.** Tell yourself every day, *"I GET to do this and live my dream of becoming the best doctor I can possibly be!"*

**170.** Think about the patients' needs first. *(You may be tired and frustrated from all the work you must do, however, your patients need your energy and compassion to heal their suffering)*

**171.** Label all lab specimens and volunteer to bring them to the lab yourself. *(It shows that you have initiative and helps ensure that your lab samples get where they're supposed to)*

**172.** Meet the lab technicians and ask them to show you peripheral smears and other slides of interest for educational purposes. *(Being an active learner and using all of your senses will enhance your education)*

**173.** Don't "space invade" the nursing stations – be mindful of your surroundings, be unobtrusive, and be respectful. *(Even though you're still a 'student' you will benefit greatly in the future by acting like a 'professional' from Day One)*

**174.** Meet with your medical team and decide on a balanced and fair system for how you will admit new patients (*e.g. one person takes medical history, another does physical exam, or alternate full admissions, etc.*).

**175.** Treat ALL patients as **people** to be cared for – not as cases to be presented. *(Your patients are human beings – treat them with dignity, respect, and compassion)*

**Notes:**

_____

_____

_____

_____

_____

_____

_____

_____

_____

_____

_____

_____

_____

_____

_____

_____

_____

_____

_____

_____

_____

_____

_____

## Notes:

_____

_____

_____

_____

_____

_____

_____

_____

_____

_____

_____

_____

_____

_____

_____

_____

_____

_____

_____

_____

_____

_____

_____

## Notes:

_____

_____

_____

_____

_____

_____

_____

_____

_____

_____

_____

_____

_____

_____

_____

_____

_____

_____

_____

_____

_____

_____

_____

_____

## Notes:

_____

_____

_____

_____

_____

_____

_____

_____

_____

_____

_____

_____

_____

_____

_____

_____

_____

_____

_____

_____

_____

_____

## Notes:

_____

_____

_____

_____

_____

_____

_____

_____

_____

_____

_____

_____

_____

_____

_____

_____

_____

_____

_____

_____

_____

_____

_____

## Notes:

_____

_____

_____

_____

_____

_____

_____

_____

_____

_____

_____

_____

_____

_____

_____

_____

_____

_____

_____

_____

_____

_____

_____

**Notes:**

_____

_____

_____

_____

_____

_____

_____

_____

_____

_____

_____

_____

_____

_____

_____

_____

_____

_____

_____

_____

_____

_____

_____

## Notes:

_____

_____

_____

_____

_____

_____

_____

_____

_____

_____

_____

_____

_____

_____

_____

_____

_____

_____

_____

_____

_____

_____

## Notes:

_____

_____

_____

_____

_____

_____

_____

_____

_____

_____

_____

_____

_____

_____

_____

_____

_____

_____

_____

_____

_____

_____

_____

_____

**Notes:**

_____

_____

_____

_____

_____

_____

_____

_____

_____

_____

_____

_____

_____

_____

_____

_____

_____

_____

_____

_____

_____

_____

_____

# About the Author

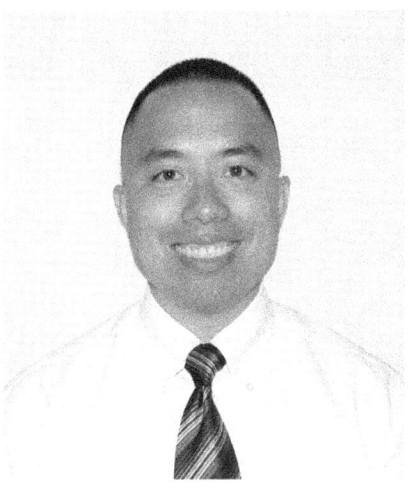

## Mel Ona, M.D., M.S., M.P.H., M.A.

Dr. Mel Ona is the author of *Changing Bodies, Transforming Lives – Your Ultimate Guide to FAD-FREE™ Fat Loss* and *"Hey, I Can See My Abs!"* He is the founder of www.MelOna.com.

Mel enjoys writing books, singing opera, playing guitar, training in mixed martial arts, lifting weights, and spending time with his loved ones and friends.

*"The good physician treats the disease; the **great** physician treats the patient who has the disease."*
– Sir William Osler